Gemma
STORY BOO

GW01079894

Some Body

Written by
Grace Godschild

Illustrated by
Harriet Stanley

Published by Rochart

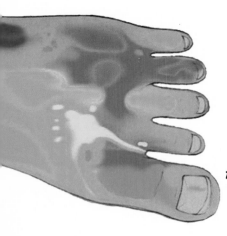

I have ten toes,

And two elbows.

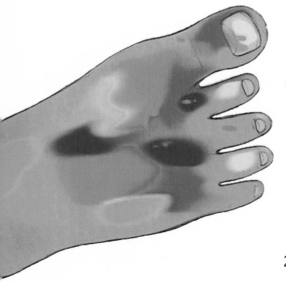

I have feet in a pair,

and lots of lovely hair.

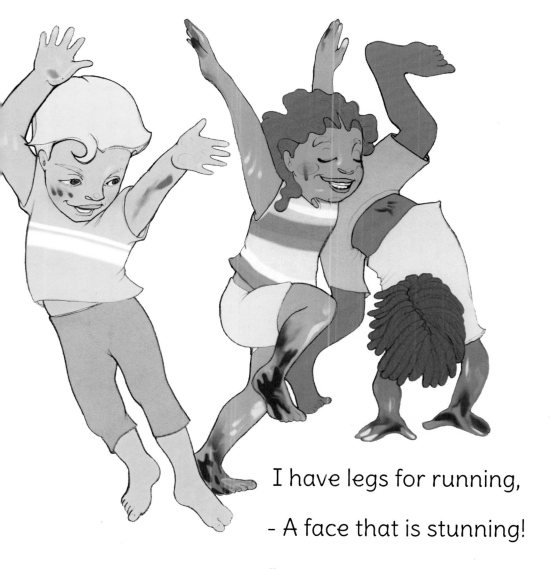

I have legs for running,

- A face that is stunning!

I have two knee caps,

and teeth without gaps,

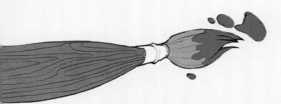

I have two very strong thighs,

and eyebrows above my eyes.

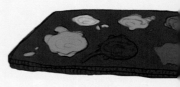

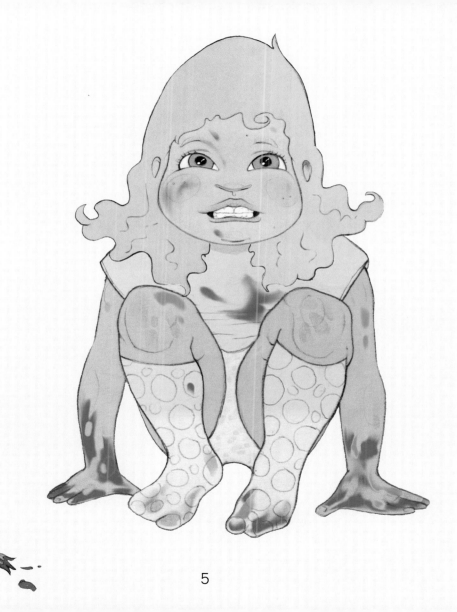

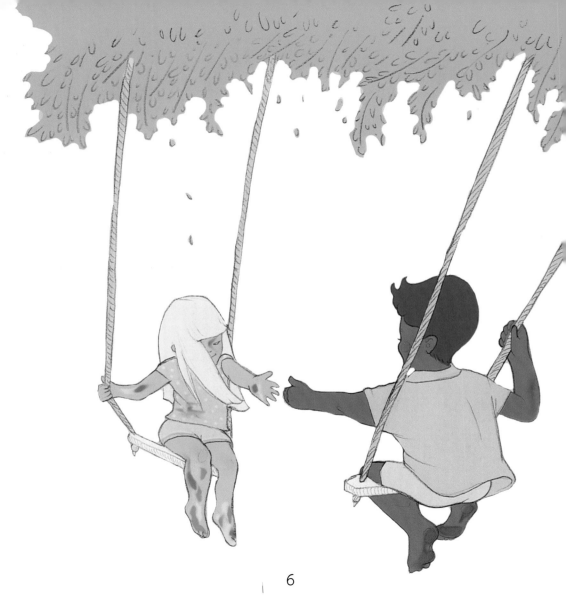

I have a bottom which can

sit on a seat,

and a tummy that's just a treat.

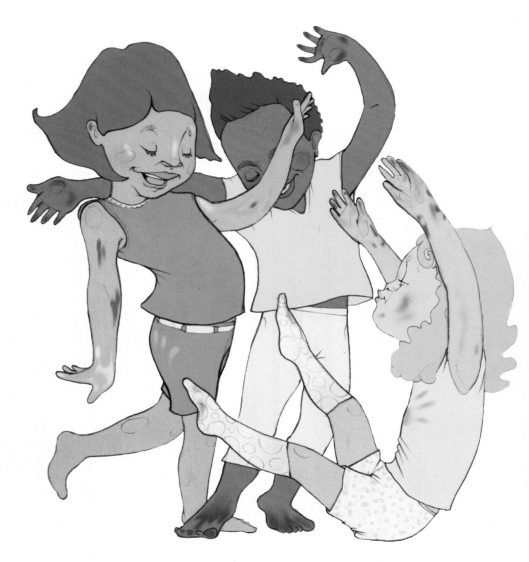

I have a useful chest,

On which my shoulders rest.

I have a back firm and strong,

And a neck slender and long.

I have two graceful arms,

Reaching down to my palms.

I have eight fingers and two thumbs,

A mouth containing all my gums.

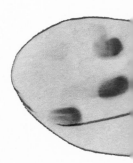

I have a brain inside my head,

And a tongue that is pinky-red.

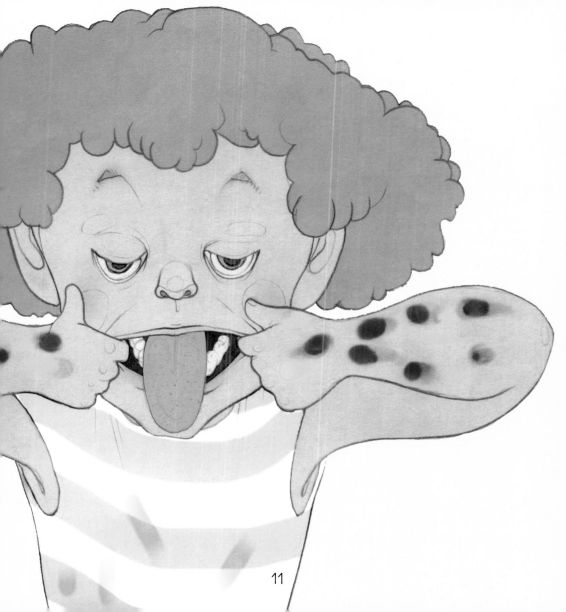

I have two eyes which open wide,

And two perfect ears at the side.

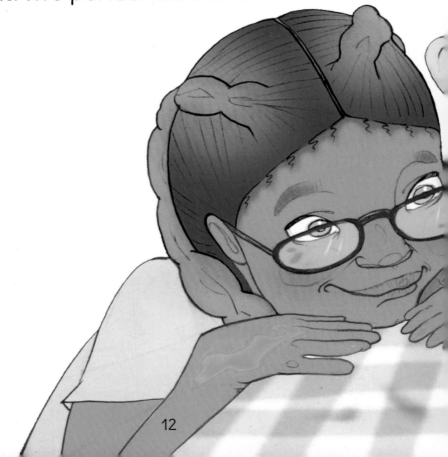

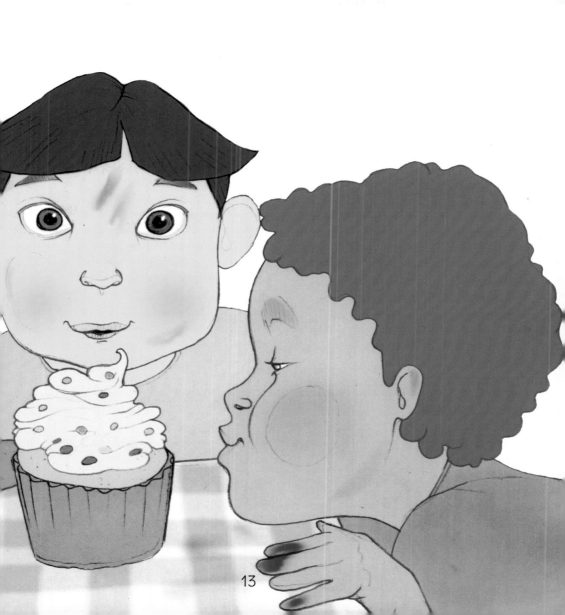

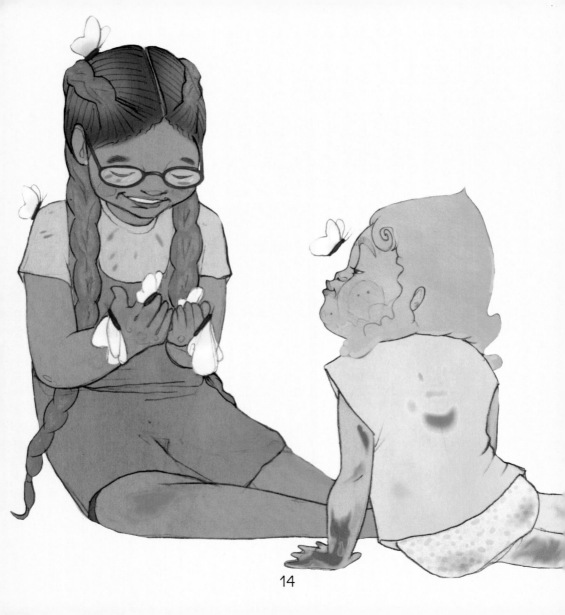

14

GOD designed my body

so well,

Thank you GOD

you are swell!

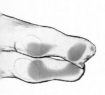

GOD designed all the outside parts,

Then came to live within my heart.

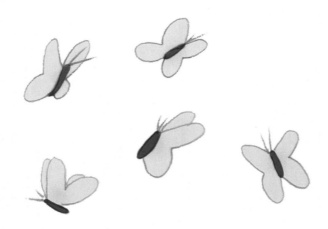

I hear you ask,

"How can this be?"

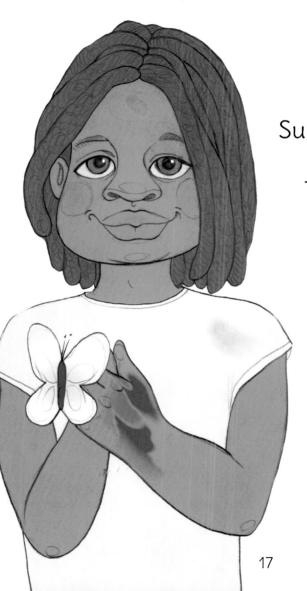

Surely it's not possible

– live within me??

But it is – because

HE is GOD

– you see!!!

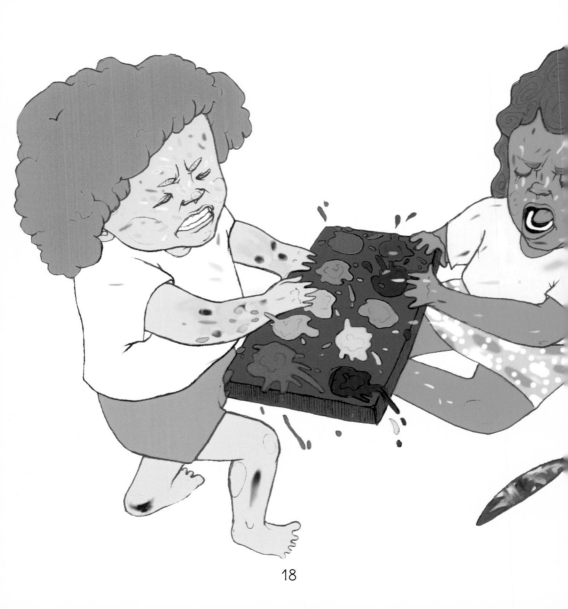

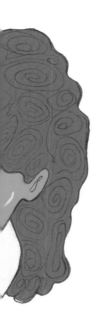

I tried not to let him in,

Because I liked all the sin.

But GOD said "No all this must stop;

It's my place – devil out you pop!"

I quite often get out of line,

But GOD says "come back – you are mine."

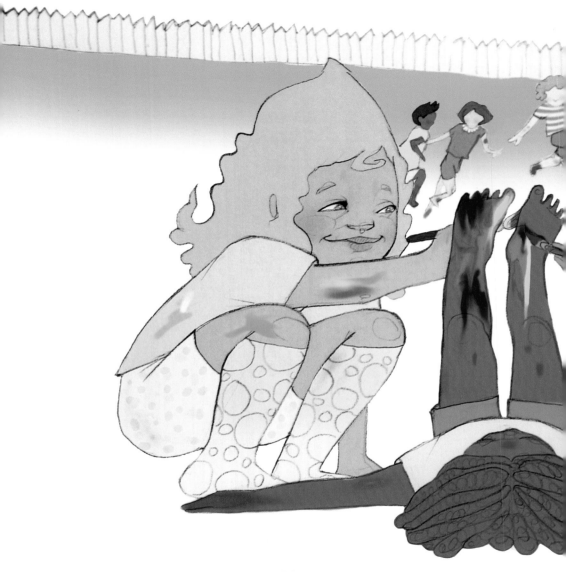

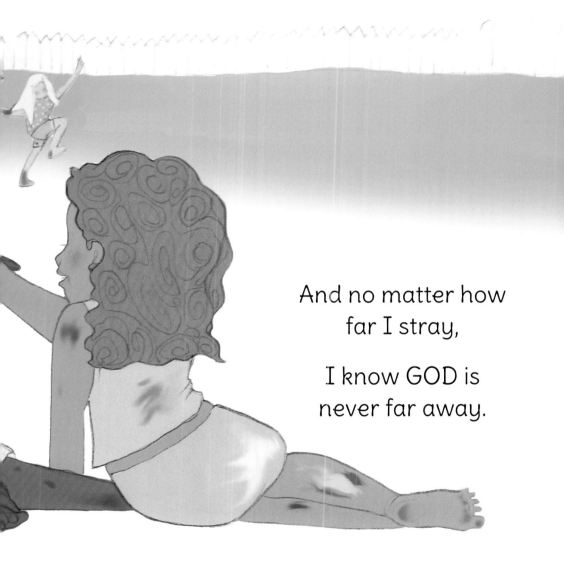

And no matter how
far I stray,

I know GOD is
never far away.

If you feel you have been away,

Come back to GOD – right now today.

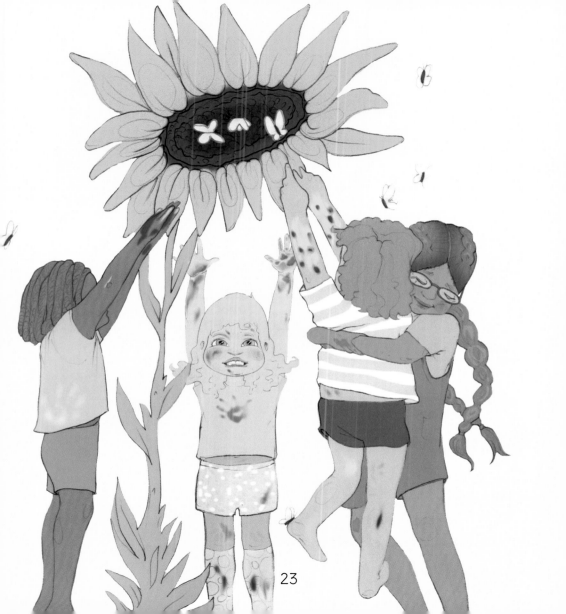

23

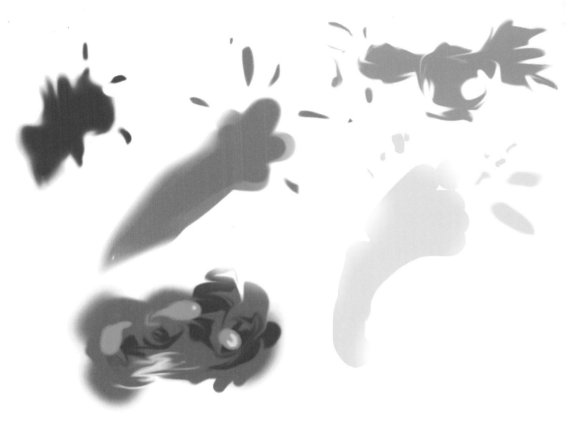

Just say "GOD I am sorry I do need you".

And it is His promise He will live within you.